Chris Brazel

Henry C

I Turn Red Flags Into Winners

Chris Brazel, Author

First published in 2022 by Chris Brazel Enterprises Pty Ltd, 5/43 Upper Brookfield Rd., Brookfield.

ISBN - 978-0-6480886-0-8

Special thanks to:

The Editor – Marcelle Charles
Formatting – Mindy Gilling
Cover and Design – Chris Brazel

You can contact the Author by email at chris@chrisbrazel.com.au. If you would like to know more about Chris Brazel's work, check out her website www.chrisbrazel.com.au

To buy further copies of the book please order through website www.chrisbrazel.com.au or email chris@chrisbrazel.

This book is dedicated to all the mums, dads and children who stepped out of the norm and into my codes.

And the biggest thank you of all to Henry C and his mum and dad.

Thank you for being part of my world.

Chris Brazel

Chapters

Introduction

This is Henry C

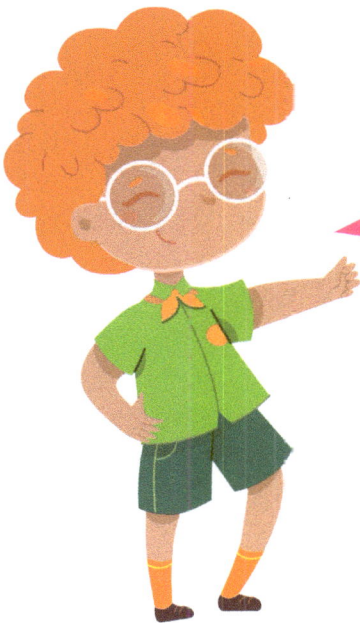

Welcome to my world

Introduction

I want to say thank you for listening to me.

I just know my story and my little tips will help you. I know because they helped me.

Sometimes in life you just have to step out of the norm. Who says the norm is right anyway?

I am so lucky to have a mum and dad like I do. They look for real solutions to real problems.

Before I learnt about my brain codes, how to work with colours and my bedroom, how to bounce a ball and that it is ok to be active, I was heading down a life of misery.

I still have those days when my mind goes at a million miles an hour. I still get the angry days and those days when I just want to yell and punch. But I get through them and, best of all, I now know the signs when they are coming so I know what to do.

If they get too bad, mum and dad help me out. I also get to work with Chris Brazel on a regular basis.

I am a member of the CB Club which is awesome in every way. The club is not just for kids who have minds that go at a million miles. Everyone is welcome in the club – all you need to qualify is to be alive. So that is pretty much anyone who can come along. Chris Brazel says you can even bring your dog along if you think you need to.

So even though I am only 8, I still need to start being responsible for me and my brain and my life now.

Trust me this works. Maybe one day we will catch up at a CB Club

Meeting, Bootcamp or Ford Car Meet when I am there with my dad. Just look for the brightest coloured car with the coolest dudes in the brightest coloured clothes.

So here is my story and my tips for you.

Henry C.

My Story

Henry C

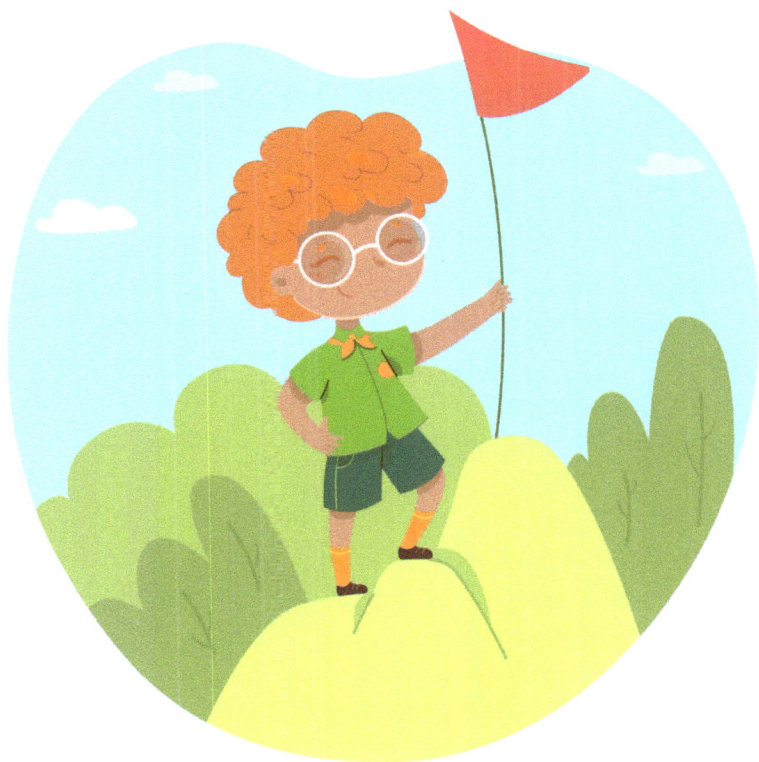

My Story

Thank God my mum is so smart and loves me to the moon and back.

The other day I was moving too much in my chair. The teacher got angry, and I could not explain that it is really hard for me to be perfectly still. It is like my brain tells me to move some part of my body.

I truly want to sit still, but this brain of mine wants something different. It is hard to explain.

Anyway, the teacher got angry again and she called my mum in to chat.

So, my mum came to school to see the teacher. I had to go along as well.

It was not a great chat and I felt so sad.

The teacher told my mum that I was not focusing on my work at school. I was fidgeting all the time and moving around. She said that when I am given tasks, I do the task but not in the way she wants it done, so she gets angry even though I finish the task and I get the answers and the sums right.

My mum was asked by the teacher to take me to one of those people who just want to talk about the problem. They make you feel so small, and I am already small, so you really do not need to be made any smaller.

Apparently, I have red flags. Now if you have a red flag in a race or out in the wind or even on a boat you are in luck and you are moving to win.

But not in this world of the mind, where they call a red flag a problem.

I don't want to be a problem. I just want to be me. Why don't they actually understand I am really an innovative kid who is bright, and I could even be like Henry Ford the guy who invented the Ford car.

My dad's into cars so maybe between the two of us we could be super inventors.

Anyway, back to the time with this counsellor

We had two sessions and it was said that I needed further help. He now wants me to go to the psychiatrist. From all the movies I have watched on TV, that is where they send mad people.

I am telling you right now – I am not mad.

I may fidget a little but that is just my body keeping up with my mind. I may be competitive but that is my inner person saying have a go and try your best.

I may think outside the square to do things in a better way, but that is great because if Edison had not thought outside the square, we would not have lights bulbs.

Anyway, Mum is doing what the experts say and we are off to the psychiatrist. We get to the psychiatrist, book in and get ready to go in for our appointment. As we sat there, I looked around. I must say it was not a great office and it did not have a great feel.

I can't say it is inviting, happy or gives you any inspiration that you are on a good thing with your mind here.

We finally get in and my mum and the psychiatrist talk about me, right in front of me. He started to ask questions. Mum answered the questions. Again, lots of chatting really about nothing.

Again, I think I got to shrink a little smaller. Lucky my mum is strong so she can re-charge me when we get out of here. I think I will be like a car with a battery. When my battery gets flat from these so called mind chats, she is going to have to plug me in and charge me up again so I can move in the world.

Listening to all of this is not great. You think your mind was a little worried before! Well, after chatting about this and really going around in circles with all these red flags, what does an 8-year-old do?

Well virtually nothing because I am 8.

But then again, I have the best mum in the world – dad is also great. They had this chat at dinner, and it is starting to look positive. Still all this red flag business, but at least I think they are coming up with solutions.

After dinner mum is on this zoom session with this lady. Super glasses I noticed at first. Then there is amazing artwork that looked so happy on the wall behind her. She was also dressed in all these bright colours. Before the meeting started, I asked mum who this cool person was.

She then explained it was Chris Brazel the world's best Brain Coder. Now she had me listening. They were going to do this Coloured Undies Meeting and talk about families and kids. She then reminded me that I had met Chris Brazel before when she came to my home before we moved from one state to another. I then remembered because she was so nice, and I remember how bright and colourful her clothes were.

She checked out my room then to make sure it was happy. We got to paint a couple of grey walls in the home to one being green and one to orange.

After her visit to the home our whole lives changed. I would call her a change maker. I had forgotten all about this fun lady until now. For a split second I had this glimmer of fate that this lady could help me. She did it once before with the whole family. Maybe mum can chat about my mind and my body and see what we can sort out.

The meeting is about to start so I am off to bed with dad and a book. As soon as the lights are out, I am going to say a little prayer. I learnt from a very young age that when we have a problem, we need to call on Blessed Mother Mary – or Our Lady to some people. She covers the world and can virtually take care of all things. So, one prayer tonight could save me, my mind and those red flags.

Well that prayer worked. I knew it would.

When I got up for breakfast the following morning, mum said that after the zoom meeting, she asked Chris Brazel about red flags and what the teacher and my counsellor plus the big guy they call the psychiatrist was saying.

Mum said Chris Brazel simply asked for my date of birth and as mum put it, "BINGO all lights were on, and we were on the new path to answers." As I said before, I love my mum. She is one smart lady.

Let's have a look at the red flags

- Being too competitive
- Moving too much
- Fidgeting all the time
- Getting angry for not getting my way

Do you want to know what Chris Brazel had to say? You see she did my Brain Codes – they connect to me, my body and the way I think about life and act and react in life.

For a start I am born with a 1/7/7/5/5 code. Yes, I know just a bunch of numbers but not to this lady. Chris Brazel has cracked the codes.

The 1 code says that I will start things but not finish them.
I will not always have focus so need to be mindful of where my focus is.
I am an innovator. I am a leader.

Lots more positive things. She had a way of mixing the positive with the energies that we needed to work on. I see a lot clearer than most.

- My eyes are important.
- My bedroom is super important.
- If I work with a ball, I will learn to be in the present moment and learn to focus.
- Martial Arts would also help me with my mind, focus and allow me to be competitive at the same time.

With the two 7s with the double 5s, I am very intelligent. I can see how things can be done in a much better way than the ways they may be doing them at the present moment.
I have this magical connection to my soul. So, I really know inside what I need. Hence the movement of my body.

With the double 5s, I need change and I need movement. At the same time, I need discipline. The main thing with the double 5s is that I need movement, hence the reason why some part of my body is moving or wants to move.

Also, with the double 5s I will have teeth problems. Which I might add is spot on. I have problems with my teeth, both upper and lower, so another spot on. I grind them all night. Not great. Can you imagine when I grow up what my wife is going to say about me. Dad is always telling me that mum keeps him awake all night. I could be doing the same thing to my wife. I want to get onto this tooth connection sooner than later and get it fixed.

With the double 7s, I can take on an emotion so when someone really says wrong things about me, I take it on, and it starts to weigh me down.

Also, with the double 7s, need alone time. I am not sulking. I just need to be alone. I do need to cry because that gets it out of me instead of holding it in.

I just need someone to come and check on me but really let me be. Once all those tears are out, I am free again. If I didn't cry and have the alone time, all that bad energy would build up and then later in life cause lots of problems.

Chris Brazel was explaining to my mum everything about me and my needs. She got the whole thing about me and my mind and how my body feels 100%. The great thing mum didn't have to say a word and I didn't have to say anything. It is like she goes inside your head and tells you everything that is going on. Even more amazing she is so spot on. 100% accurate.

You know the best thing is that she is going to show me and my mum and dad how to work with my brain to get this mind working in perfect harmony.

Perfect harmony so I get to be ME, and I get to grow up allowing my talents and innovation come to the forefront instead of those mind doctors just giving me a pill. Once again, I have to say I am so proud of my mum for standing up for me and no pills.

Chris Brazel is coming over to look at my room and we are going to work together. I am going to learn the Bounce 2 Ball and You programme. I am also going to enter into the Bounce 2 Championships. I am going to learn about colour, my mind, meditations, working with a ribbon and all amazing things.

Best of all I now have someone who totally understands my brain and how my mind works so as a team, along with my mum and dad, I get to grow up and take my part in the world exactly how I am meant to. If I was simply to pop a pill every day, I would be crushing ME. I would be moving into a definition of a puppet. Never being able to pull my own strings.

But not closing on that sad note. I am going to be a top Innovator for the world. If Henry Ford can come up with the car – I can go one better. Not sure what, but watch this space over the years. If all of a sudden, you hear or watch on TV that this amazing cool dude has invented some form of transport that is out of this world, then Ah! that would be ME, the almighty Henry C.

Henry C

Colour and my Mind

Henry C

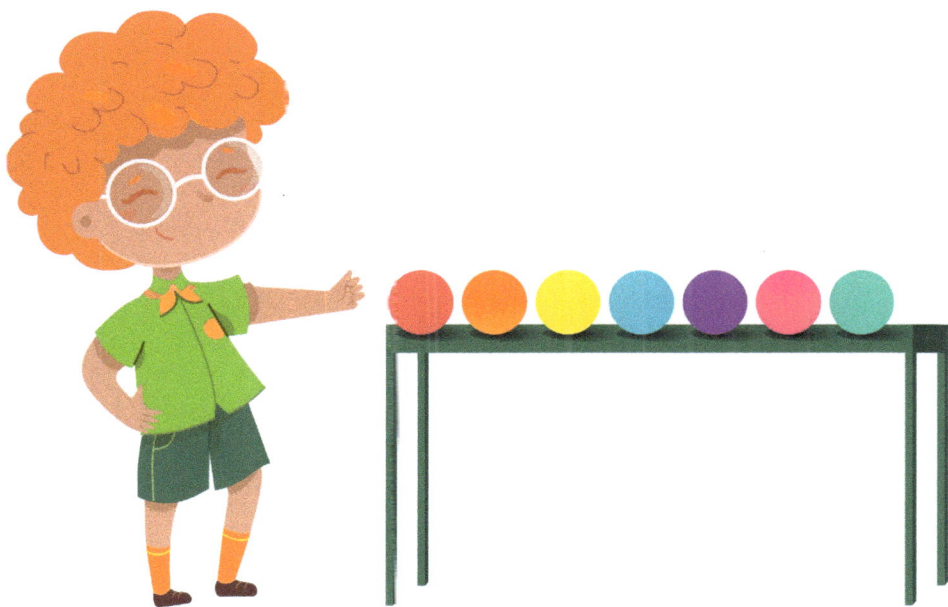

Colour and My Mind

Learning about colour is awesome. It is like your own private weapon. When you choose a colour that means you are making a choice through your mind. When you make a choice through your mind and you know the purpose of the colour as to what you want in life, that is when you feel in control.

Every colour has a special energy to work with. Every code that you have for your brain has a colour to work with. It is so easy, you are heading into an exam, you think you know the answers and it will be ok.

Well, you simply put on the red undies and, as you do, you tell your mind that you are going to pass your exams today and that you will remember all the things you need to remember and will get what you can right. You give your mind confidence that everything is going to be ok.

It is not about just wearing red undies. You can wear a red t-shirt or have a red pen or have strawberries for breakfast that day.

The fun part about colour is you can use it in so many ways.

- Your undies come first
- Your clothes
- Your shoes
- Your food
- Your room
- Your books
- Your library bag and heaps more ways. I bet you can think of a few yourself

Did you notice what I was trying to tell you in all the ways you can wear colour?

The" your" is you. You step into the power.

You may have to teach your mum about a colour or two but by now you have this book so your mum is already onto it and will definitely help you out. If she is like my mum, they love you so much and just want your mind to be right.

Have you seen how much black clothing there is in the world? I was in one of the shops the other day and saw this black jumper with these weird sad drawings on the front. Don't these designers know what they are doing to us kids' minds. The only thing I can say is that, if they are designing like that, then their mind is like that.

You would never see Chris Brazel design anything like that.

I now do not wear black unless it is a necessity at school or karate event. I wear all the colours that I want to feel each day.

I have a little list for you below, but if you want to know more, then just spend one day with Chris Brazel and you will know the magic of colours and colour combinations. Here are the colours I know that I can share with you to help you right away:

Red

Confidence, focus, proud

Orange

When you need change or want to change something

Yellow

The happy colour, it picks you up. It helps you get clarity for your mind. It is a knowing. When you know things, you can be confident, just like the sun that comes up every morning and goes down every afternoon. That is a knowing that everything will be ok.

Green

I love the green. It connects to love, being able to grow just like the trees and the plants in the world. When you connect to green, and you think of nature you know that someone up there can make anything happen.

Blue

Great to help you communicate and feel the emotions you are feeling.
Too much blue can make you feel too emotional, and you can feel like you are drowning – not great.

So, you need to work on the right amount of blue. Now this is light blue I am talking about.

Navy

A strong blue that helps you take responsibility for your life.
It helps you speak from within.
It helps you connect to your soul.
We all have a soul you know, just like we have a heart.

Purple

Belief in yourself. It can also help you to find the knowledge you need. Chris Brazel said that when you need to face the truth about something then have purple and white together.

She has some great things in purple and white.   Check out her website.

White

White helps you with clarity and structure. So, you need some white in your life. White is also great to go with your colours

For example, if you have a red jumper and you have white writing on it such as, "I am Awesome" then that is really getting through to your mind what you want to be and feel.

Pink

Pale pink helps to keep you calm. I know most boys don't wear a lot of pink, but you may have a sister who you can help out. Or maybe your mind needs to calm the farm so you could work with the pink.

Hot Pink

This is a step up from the pale pink but not as strong as the red. Still a great colour for confidence when you don't want to be too out there.

Grey

Well, I am afraid that grey is grey. It is neither one thing nor another. Who wants to be in no man's land not being able to make a decision?

Black

You have to be very careful with this colour. Chris Brazel won't wear anything that is black. The children who work really close with her and are real winners in life and feel great about life do not wear black in their clothing either.

Black shoes will be ok – I have checked because they are touching the ground and grounding you.

You just don't put black around your heart space or your head space.

So, my line in the sand goes here today. Black is out for me and my mind in clothes. I will allow myself black shoes to work on my grounding, knowing that I have made the choice about the black in the right way.

I will use a black belt in karate as that is a special thing where I am learning the rules of martial arts.

Brown

Brown can make you feel bogged down. A little brown on your shoes is great as it will ground you. So, a colour to be careful of and wear the right way to the way your mind is behaving.

There is so much more you can learn about colour, but I will leave that to you and whether you want to learn more. The more you learn the more you take control of your mind and are the driver of the car of your life.

By the way I haven't told dad yet, but I am aiming for a Porsche. A Porsche Boxster like Chris Brazel drives. I went for a drive with her. She promised me I could go for a drive if I cleaned up my room.

"Oh man it was awesome!"

Give colour a try, it can't hurt you and you never know you might just start to feel great like me.

Keep reading. I still have more to tell you.

Henry C.

My Bedroom and My Mind

Henry C

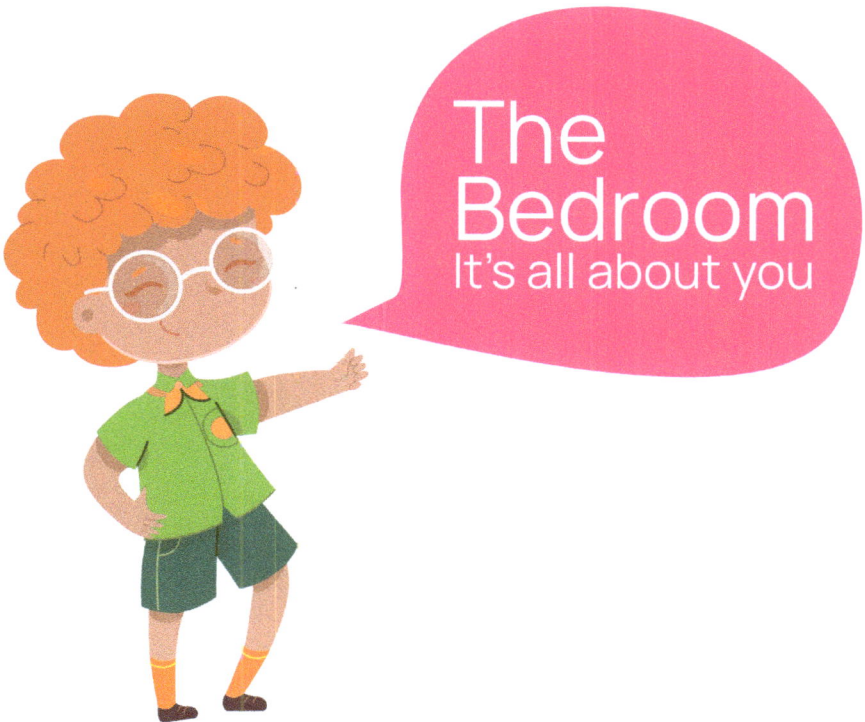

The
Bedroom
It's all about you

My Bedroom and My Mind

Who would have thought that your bedroom is a duplicate of your mind and how you are feeling and thinking about life?

Well today Chris Brazel comes for the inspection. I have made sure it is all neat and tidy. I think mum is more worried about the inspection than me.

I figure she is just going to say move that, change this and really at the end of the day she is coming to help, not hinder so what is there to be afraid of?

So, do you want to know what she said?

She stood at the door and looked in. She was so quiet. She just looked at my room.

I looked at her face to see what she was thinking, but she does not give anything away.

Finally, she spoke and here is the diagnosis and my thoughts as we went through the room.

My Bedroom

First, I have her comments then my thoughts:

My room felt empty - I would agree to that.
The bed was in the middle and wrong type of bed – Yay, I have been telling my parents that.
The quilt is too grown up – Yes, I would agree to that.
Your shoes, on the shoe rack look like you are going uphill – I didn't think of that but now she mentioned the fact, I can totally see what she means.

They were the main things that were wrong. She was so spot on and exactly how I was feeling as well.

What was Right?

As you look into my room I had my books – great – tick.
Above my books I had one of her special pictures. She was pretty proud of that. She had forgotten that she had given an original to my mum years ago.
The way I had my clothes in the wardrobe – great – tick.
I had lots of coloured shirts – great- tick.
I had a selenite lamp – super – tick.

What are We going to Change?

Moving the bed into the control position so I have view of the window and the doors.
Change the quilt on my bed. Chris Brazel is actually going to help me design my own quilt.
Place one of my favourite Pokémon pictures on the wall.
Fix my shoes so it does not feel I am going uphill and hard work.
Add another stand for my books so I can gain more knowledge.
I can just see my room now. No longer like an adult's room with a big bed where you feel you can swim in it. I am going to have a real kid's room that looks and feels like a kid's room. I am only 8 years old so need a room that resembles an 8-year-old. I have a bit of living to do yet.

I learnt a lot today, so I am going to share the tips with you.

Tips for Your Bedroom

Make sure your bed is in the control position. The control position is when you have sight of the door and the windows.

Never have your bedhead on the wall where the door is as that is the fear position. That means you will feel frightened. You don't know what is going on and you can't see who is coming and what is happening.

The pictures on the wall are really important as they give triggers to your mind. For example, Chris Brazel told me about this little boy who had a picture of an Indian sitting on a horse ready to spear a fish. A bit scary to wake up to each day.

The colours in your bedroom are really important. You should have the colours that match your codes.

I found out that too much blue can make you too emotional. If you don't know what that word means – in short you just want to cry a lot and be sad.

Definitely no black walls or grey walls.
No black, grey, or brown quilts
If you have a 1 code as your natural code, you need to be able to see out the window.

One rule when you are in the CB club is that you make your bed each day.

Chris Brazel is a little easier on the other rules, but no getting out of making your bed.

She says that if you come into your room and all you see is a messy bed, then you start to get a messy head.

Put your shoes away neat and tidy.

Now I have a 7 code so shoes are really important for me to look after.
I now know to put my shoes neat and tidy in my cupboard.

I face them out, so they feel free.
I never face them into the wall as that makes you feel you have obstacles in your way.

Trust me there is a bit to earn but once you get it, then life is great.

As I said before, I still have those days when I get angry. My head is going at a million miles, I want to punch the wall, but I have the tools to get through it.

When you have the toolbox of tools, then like any good car, you can keep it running smoothly.

Mum bought one picture I love which Chris Brazel designed and it is a picture of a white horse with a little boy snuggled up beside. It feels so good. You feel so safe. When you look at it, you just know that there is always someone there to take care of you.

I don't have a 9-brain code but if you do, one thing will be important and that is to toss out or hand over to charity the clothes you no longer wear or use.

If you learn to do this when you are young, then it won't be so hard when you get older.

You see, with a 9 brain code holding on and not letting go, it can be a problem a little later on, so the earlier we get to deal with our mind, the easier life will be when we get older.

There are of course some things you can keep for a million years. Well by that I mean all your life. They are the special treasures that mean a lot to you.

Just make sure that you don't think every single thing is a treasure. This is when you have so much there is just no space in your room.

I saw one kid's room recently and there were so many stuffed toys it was a wonder he could get to his bed.

The curtains are important.
Your desk is also important if you do your homework in your room.
There are lots of ways to design your room.

I have given you a few tips. The best idea would be to check out Chris Brazel's website and YouTube where you will learn lots. Come to a bootcamp or simply get her to come and check out your room.

I did hear about one scary room a parent designed for her daughter.

Here it is – can you just imagine how this little girl felt. No wonder, as Chris Brazel said, she didn't want to sleep in her room.

Are you ready?

You stand at the door, and you look in.

On the wall on the right and I mean a whole wall, there is this wallpaper of dead trees -all black dead trees like they had been burnt in a fire.
Then in the middle of the forest of dead burnt trees is this bird with its wings spread out flying towards you. Well, it looks like the bird is flying towards you. Chris Brazel says it feels like the bird is saying, "Get me out of here."

Well, the mum could not see the problem with the wallpaper. Apparently, it was designer wallpaper. That simply means the mum paid way too much for the messy sad thoughts of another person.

Then it gets better, or I should say worse. On her bedspread there is one of the same dead burnt trees on a white quilt. So, if the little girl didn't get enough of the sad scary stuff off the wall, she had to sleep under the quilt of a night.

No wonder she was anxious, sad and crying that she didn't want to sleep in her room. The mum thought she was just being anxious. As they say these days without any thought to us kids, we have a mental problem. I may be only eight but even I know why the little girl gets scared and anxious in her room.

Anyway, I asked Chris Brazel if the mum changed the wallpaper.

Chris Brazel said that she just left the mum with a plan and had not heard what happened.

I am going to make sure when I get all this finished, I go and give my mum a huge hug. I know she has got my back.

This is Henry C over and out to the next chapter.

Henry C

Bounce a Ball and Change Your Thoughts

Henry C

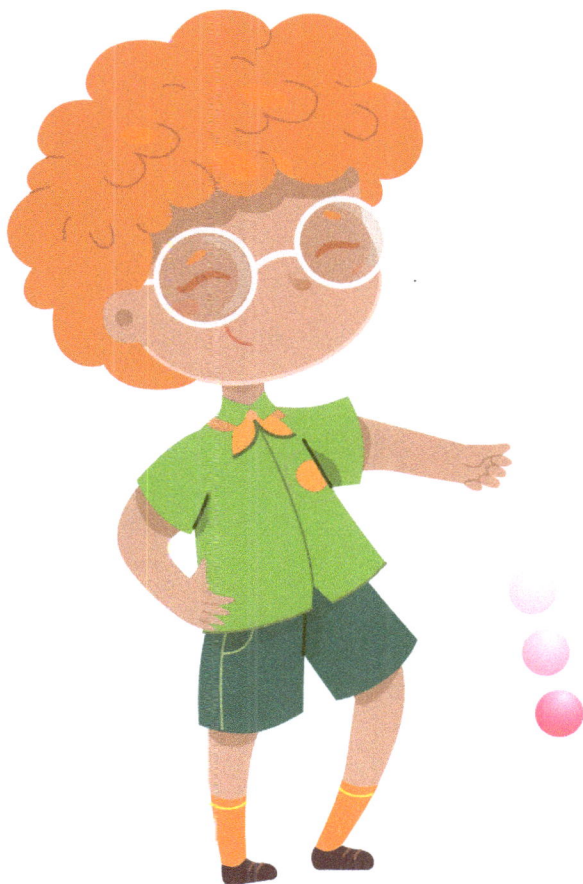

Bounce a Ball and Change Your Thoughts

I must say of all the tips Chris Brazel has given me this one is the best.

I love it. I get to play at the same time as sorting out my mind.

In fact, this exercise works so fast I am over the mind worry and mind games in seconds.

You see, with my brain codes, focus is important as well as concentration. Also, counting the bounces gives me a starting point and finishing point so I get confident that I can do things.

With the ball I learnt that when I bounce the ball I am connecting to my mind through movement and my hands. When I add a special ball colour, that makes the exercise stronger and more powerful.

Let me explain what I mean.

When I need to be confident, I work with a red ball.

If something has happened at school during the day, my mind is still trapped there, and my mind won't let it go. The story starts to happen, and I get all these thoughts messing up my head. I get my orange ball and bounce it to the floor or ground with words Chris Brazel has taught me. Orange means change with choice and releasing.

Chris Brazel taught me the words that go with the bouncing of my orange ball.

What ever happened yesterday, is all gone now. What ever happened before, that is worrying me, is all gone now.

I have to bounce the ball 9 times which is closing a door, then I toss it up in the air and sing out, "Everything is great again."

Normally by the 3rd time I have done this exercise, my mind is fine.

If I am worried about my exams or having to go somewhere new, I take my red ball and toss it to the wall. Depending on what I need to happen, I say some words.

For example: If I am worried about my exam that I am not going to pass, I take my red ball for confidence, and I bounce it to the floor and say, "I can pass my exam."

I then take my red ball and toss it to the wall (that means I am breaking through) and say, "I am passing my exam."

Then I toss it up in the air and say, "I have passed my exam."

It is so clever. You try it and see.

There are a whole heap of ball exercises to work with – check out the Bounce 2 Bal Programme and give them a go. You can even join the Bounce 2 Championships. I might see you there one day.

You learn the difference between working with the left hand, then working with the right hand.

Another great one when you are feeling sad is to face a wall and work with your left hand tossing the ball to the wall, then your right hand, then alternate left and right hand.

For this you should work with a yellow or orange ball. It is good if you have a collection of balls. That way you have everything covered no matter how your mind feels.

The best is the Bounce 2 handball game. You play on a table like table tennis but instead of a bat you use your hands. You can also work through to championships, so you can see how good you can get.

There is no fighting, as the rules are simple. One bounce either side of the net.

If the ball goes off the table, it is out and hand over.

First person to 21 wins.

I am going to practise so I can play in the Australian Bounce 2 Championships.

How cool would it be to be the first 8-year-old Bounce 2 Handball Champion?

Henry C.

Climb a Mountain or Stairs and Conquer a Thought

Henry C

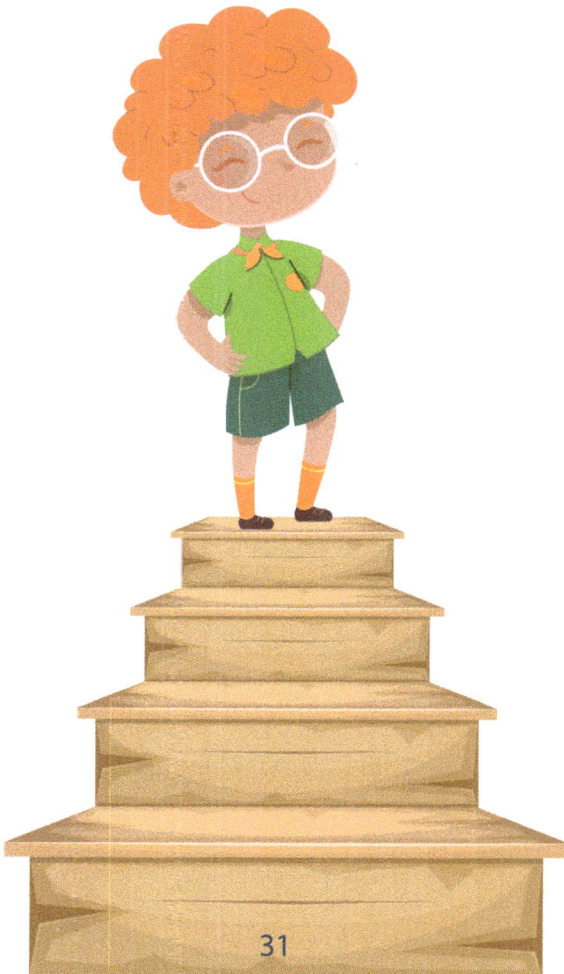

Climb a Mountain or Climb a set of Stairs and Conquer a Thought

This is an awesome way to train your brain to move from sad to confident, or to move from scared to being strong. You are training your brain that you can do this.

Take your mum or dad along as it is awesome to see how their mind changes at the same time.

I take my mum. It is great. She needs to change a few things in her life, so we are kind of working together to create a great life and manifest our new home.

My mum is also joining me for the Bounce 2 dance moves, and we have heaps of fun with the Handball Bounce 2 Game.

The main thing with the hill or mountain is that before you start to climb to the top you have to know what you want to conquer or what you want to achieve. You set your intention at the bottom of the hill and off you go to the top. As you go up you repeat the words to your goals over and over in your mind.

You can either say it over and over in your mind as you go up, or you can say it at the start, climb a bit, have a rest, say it over again either loud or just in your head, go a bit further and do the same thing.

I am getting fitter and mum, well she is working on getting fitter. I am lucky she needs a few breaks so the way we work it as a team we kick off and go a little way. She has a rest and I get to say my words over in my head. We just keep doing the same thing until we get to the top.

The key is you have to go to the top of the hill or the mountain. You never stop halfway as that means you have told your mind you only half do things.

If you have a 1 brain code, it is even more important to have a starting point and a finishing point.

I like to wear my red undies or my red shirt when I do these exercises. The red keeps me confident and my mind on track.

Make sure you use the right words. Ask your mum for help if you need any.

Climbing Stairs to Conquer a Thought.

Stairs are also great to work with to train your brain.

You do the same thing. You set an intention at the bottom of the stairs then you climb to the top one step at a time. Make sure you do not miss any steps. The key is not missing steps and going to the top. It does not matter how long it takes. What matters is that you start and take one step at a time until you get to the top.

You can kick off with just a few steps and get fitter then go for more and more stairs as you get fitter.

This feels so good in your mind. You feel amazing like you have conquered the world.

You are the totally training your brain to what you want, and you are conquering the thoughts that are not good for your mind and putting in place the feelings you want to have.

I have one extra tip for you.

If you get up early and do your hill or stair climbing at sunrise you are starting new things.

If you need to close a door, then you can go at sunset which is about closing doors. Just as the sun comes up, so new things can come into your life.

Just as the sun goes down, you are closing doors and letting go of things in your life.

Sometimes it is nice just to get up and watch a sunrise or a sunset.

When you sit there, just be still and be at peace. It is a time when I take my special crystal with me and hold it in my hand and, as I watch either the sunrise or the sunset, my mind relaxes and I feel great. I feel at peace with the world and life.

Give this a go – challenge your mum or dad to go with you.

A bit of a challenge any time is good for the mind and soul.

Henry C

Make a Deal With My Mind

Henry C

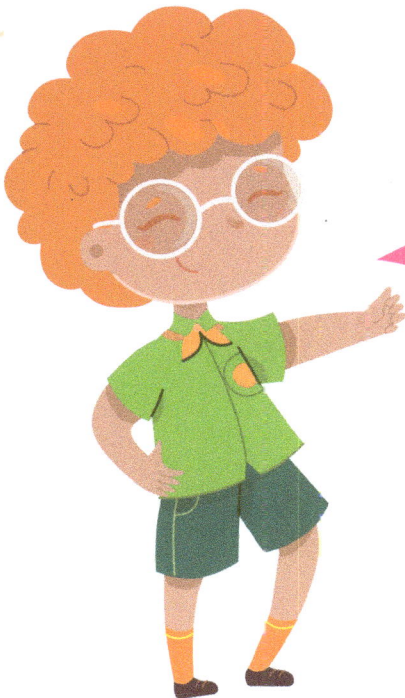

Make a deal with your mind

Make a Deal with My Mind

With my double 5 code I need freedom.

I will move and I will fidget. So how do I conquer these little things that my mind wants but may not always be what my teacher or older people want?

So here is my plan that Chris Brazel designed and taught to me.

- I have a routine.
- I make a deal with my mind.
- I make a commitment to do something which leads me to doing what I want.
- I co-operate with my mum who totally understands me.
- I communicate to my teacher in a way that she understands.
- I move from chasing what I need.
- I stand in my power and attract to me what I need

The deal with my mind is such an awesome way to work. As soon as Chris Brazel told me I knew we could do this.

So here are a few tips if you are like me:

I take a worry stone and put it in my pocket to use at school and especially in the classroom.
When my body wants to move it is easy, as I can move my fingers with my worry stone. When it is in my pocket, nobody even sees it only me.

The clue is to tell my mind that it is ok. When I get to recess, I am going to move this body heaps and heaps. In the meantime, it will be just my fingers.

I learnt that the hand is about receiving. When I work with my hand with my stone, I am receiving what the mind wants to do but I am not being in trouble from my teacher for moving my body too much.

The fingers, I have found out, all have different mind connections as well so when I use my thumb on my right hand, I am being flexible with not moving with my body in the classroom. If I move my thumb on my left hand, I am giving myself belief this is going to work.

Even your right and left hand have mind connections. This is such an awesome way to work.

The way I am going to co-operate with my mum is not get angry because she is not listening to me but have a plan. We both know that when I am starting to get angry, we sit with a cup of tea which I know she loves, and I just have water as I love that, and we will talk it out.

She has also learnt that, when I get angry, it is often because of having so many emotions going around in my head that I don't know which one to deal with. It is like too much in my head, so Chris Brazel has taught me that it is ok to take time out in my room and just relax. Mum knows that I am just taking time out and that she does not need to keep pestering me to see if I am ok. I just need my space to calm my mind down the way I now know.

Mum has explained to my dad that he does not need to ask me a million times what is wrong. I don't know what is wrong because my mind is going in too many directions.

If I can be quiet in my room, I can sort it out. When parents and teachers keep at you that is when you get angry because it is just another voice in your head.

If the problem is really bad Chris Brazel has taught me the Bounce 2 Ball and You exercises which are great. Because of my 1 natural code, the moment I work with a ball my mind calms down and I have a new focus.

I have different coloured balls for different feelings.

So, now instead of getting angry and blowing up at mum or anyone else, I have a plan that I can work with because you know when the kettle within you is about to boil.

If by any chance the anger happens at school, well I will take my ball and practise there. The best thing about the Bounce 2 Ball exercises is that you can totally take control of the mind and you can do it anywhere.

My teacher and me – well that is another story. Not sure she believes in all of this, so I am going to have to toe the line a little more there.

I now have a watch which I love, and I set myself time limits to keep her happy. I also try to just do it her way. I can be an innovator when I get home. Even if the way she is teaching, to my mind, is out of date. I know with some adults they can only do one thing one way, not like us people who want to invent new ways all the time.

Working with my dad – well that is going to be easy as I have told him I have the number 1 natural brain code like Henry Ford and my dad is so into the Ford Car I am sure we can come up with a plan with parts and cars.

Chris Brazel has taught me that when you chase you are always on the run. Your mind does not get to rest and know what it is like to have what you want.

When you stand in your power and you tell your mind what to do and not let the mind tell you, then that is when you feel so powerful.

Words and actions are the best way to take over the chasing of the mind and to stand in your power.

I hope these little tips of mine have helped you.

You should come to one of our bootcamps or school camps or better still ask your mum if you can become a member of the CB Club. You get to learn so much and it is fun at the same time.

This is Henry C onto the next chapter.

Words, Ask for Help, Ask a Question

Henry C

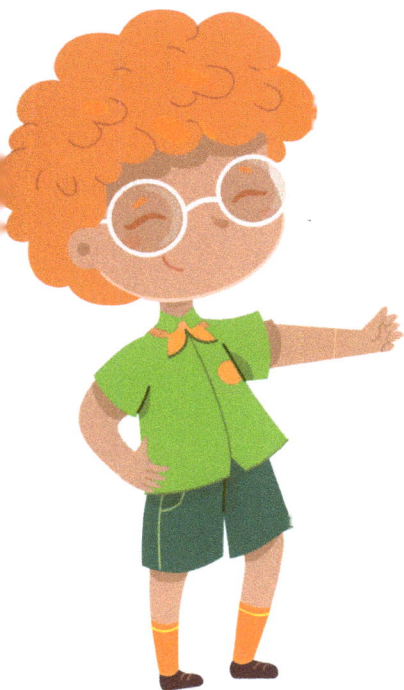

Knowledge is the key

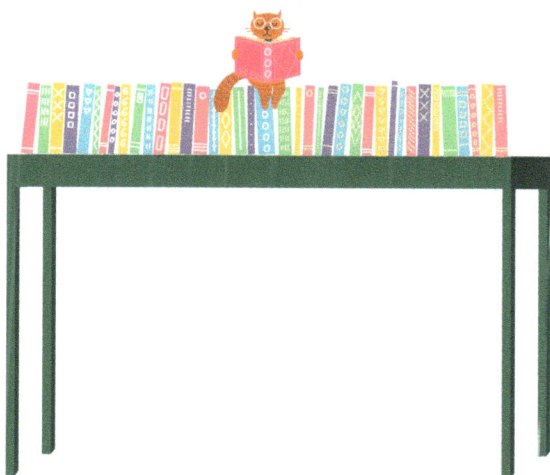

Get the Answers, Ask the Question, Ask for Help

You know I have been learning things the hard way all my life and I am only eight.

It is like I have to cause a problem, be in the problem and guess what, I then go and learn that same problem again.

Do you do the same thing? Like you get into trouble for something, then the next day you do the same thing, so you get in trouble all over again.

I used to get lots of emotions and lots of going around in circles with my mind.

Always in trouble and nobody really understanding me and my mind.

My mind used to just go places and I could not control it so I would get angry, upset, annoyed and nothing seemed to work.

Well, that was until Chris Brazel came along.

You spend one hour with her or go to one of her bootcamps and courses and man, your life kicks over like a new battery in a Ford Mustang.

Let me show you a few tips. The first one is asking.

If you don't ask, then you don't know as she says.

She told me about this boy, who is now a man. Well, he is 28 I suppose that is a man. Let's just say he is older than me and not as old as my dad.

He is now the "Know-it-all-King."

Chris Brazel told me that when the Know-it-all King was 8 years old just like me, he would go to bed of a night and be scared all night that an asteroid might come through his bedroom window and blow him up. You can actually listen to his story on our special podcasts.

He would hide under the bed clothes and start to pray that he would get through the night, and he would be ok.

Well, if you listen to his podcast with Chris Brazel, you will hear how he suffered night in and night out until he grew up.

He will tell you that now he knows that the probability of it happening is like 1 in 500,000.

What he wished he had done was chat with his mum about what he was scared of then she could have given him the answers so he would not need to be afraid.

After hearing this story, I have made a decision that when I am afraid, I am just going to ask my mum or my dad.

There is nothing wrong in asking. If you don't ask you don't know.

I don't want to be the Know-it-all King and have to wait until I am 28 to stop being afraid.

It was like he was carrying all this weight for years which he didn't need to carry.

You see when you are afraid or scared of something there is always an explanation or a reason. So, if you sort it out with your parents when it happens, things will work out.

If you just sit on it or hide under the covers it just gets worse.

With my mind codes I do get a little anxious. I worry a little as well.

Now I know how my mind works and my mum and dad know I will ask the questions.

You see I would worry if they were away and not at home. I would worry that they were not going to pick me up on time. I would worry if I was by myself.

Now I ask the question. What time will you be picking me up? Mum tells me the exact time.

Chris Brazel has taught her that my mind goes into a panic when I don't know things. So, before she used to say she would pick me up after school, which that could be any time after school. Now she tells me and in her exact words "Henry C, I am picking you up at 3.45pm." There are no grey areas there. I have a watch so I know by the time I get out of class and walk to the place where parents pick you up, she will be there at 3.45pm. She is never late.

Before I would go to the spot to be picked up, I would not see her, so my mind started to panic, as she had said she was picking me up after school. Well school had finished, and she was not there. So where was she?

Chris Brazel explained to my mum the difference in how my mind works in comparison to other kids.

She explained that it is important to give me facts. When I have facts then I know what is happening. She also gives me a back-up plan. So, between the facts and the back-up plan my mind is fine. Well 98% of the time. So much better than 10% of the time.

There is always going to be that little 2% of worry and that's ok as I have the back up plans to cover that 2% when it happens.

The best advice I can give you is getting those brain codes done. They will explain everything about you.

The other important thing in this chapter I need to teach you is the words you use each day.

There is a lot of difference between words.

Let me show you:

When you keep saying "can't" then you can't.
If you keep saying "maybe", then it will be a maybe.
If you keep saying "should" then you should.

Words are the king of the mind. When you learn the right words to say and write, you get to power the mind. Let's use the car again as an example. If you put water into a car instead of petrol the motor stops and you go nowhere – the engine is ruined.

Now if you put petrol into the car, it goes.

If you happen to put the top grade petrol in the car, it goes like a well-tuned Ford Mustang.

It is the same with your mind. If you speak words that are bad, then it is like putting water into the car. Eventually your mind will not work.

If you use the right words for the mind, it is like putting petrol into the car. It can move.

If you use great words for the mind, it is like putting top grade petrol into a car. You move with power and force.

Let me give you an example:

You say each day, "I can't do this." You are telling your mind you can't do it.

If you say each day, "I will give this a go," you are telling your mind you are going to try.

If you say each day, "I can do this," you have just put the top words into mind like you have put the top grade petrol into the car.

What you tell your mind each day is how your mind will work.

I do hope I have not made this chapter too hard.

Let's go over it again:

- Ask for help when you need it.
- If you are frightened of something, ask the question whether you should be worried or not.
- The words you say each day are your mind power. Make sure you use the top words.

Our word list -what is in and what is out. Are you ready?

Out
- Can't
- Should
- Maybe

In

- Can
- Will
- I am

Well on to another chapter. I do trust mum and dad are helping you with this book.

I think it is just as much for them as you.

Henry C.

My Secret Weapons.
Nothing like Silent Power

Henry C

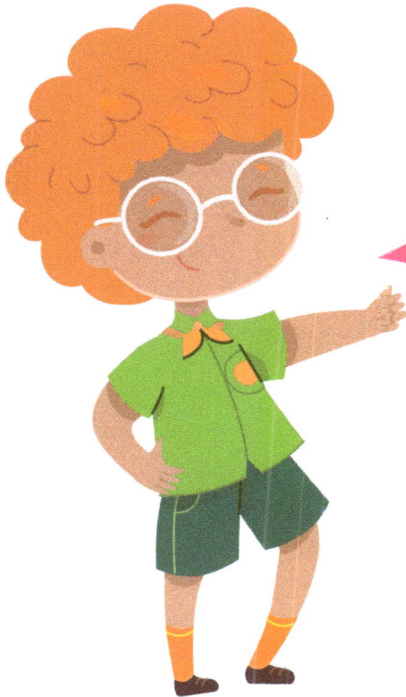

My Secret Weapons.
Nothing like Silent Power

A kid always needs that secret weapon - well, not like a machine gun.   My secret weapons are my power switches for my mind.

It is like when your mobile phone battery is running low and about to stop, you plug it into the power point, and you get going again.

It is like your mind when it starts to go flat, and you get sad, or it goes haywire, you need to have the switch to the power to fix it.

Chris Brazel has taught me a few so I am going to share them with you.

The Figure Eight

Yep, who would have thought that walking or drawing a figure 8 would help your head?

So, how does it help your head? The figure eight connects to balance. The energy of the number eight is control, timing and it is a very karmic number.

I am sure you know what control is by now.

I am also sure you know about timing. You know when the teacher says you have 5 minutes to finish. She does not mean 10 minutes or 1 hour. She means 5 minutes.

Well karmic is easy – what you give out is what you get back.

If I throw a ball really hard and fast at you, then it is more than likely you are going to throw it back at me really hard.

If I drop all my things on the floor, then the karma of that is that they stay there.

If I say nasty things to someone, then often they are going to say nasty things back to me.

So, when you decide you need to activate your secret power – your secret weapon for your mind - you walk a figure eight.

Chris Brazel has a video so you can watch her, or come to one of our courses.

Here is how it goes.

You know things in your head are not going great, so you make a decision. It's time to switch the power on.

You tell your mind that you are the one in control and you walk the figure eight. You can do it anywhere. Sometimes I even skip it, so it looks in the playground as if I am having fun.

If I am somewhere I can't go and walk my figure eight, such as in the movies or sitting in a bus, then I draw my figure eight.

I still have to tell my mind that I am flicking the switch, and that I am taking over and being in control. Then I draw my figure eight. I have a special CB notebook that Chris Brazel designed that I carry. You can get a small one or a medium size one.

I caught dad the other day walking a figure eight in the back yard. I didn't say anything. I just watched. I figured that his mind was not where he wanted it to be.

You see this figure eight secret weapon and flicking the switch works for everyone.

Tip Number 2

Crystals

As I mentioned in the previous chapter crystals are awesome.

Every crystal has a special energy the same as every number has an energy and every colour has an energy. The power for the mind is knowing the codes of it all.

With the crystals, as I mentioned previously, you can massage them in your pocket when in class when you feel like fidgeting and moving your body. Nobody knows because your hands are in your pocket.

Hands are about receiving. So, when you massage a certain crystal in your hand you have made a choice to help your mind be ok and that you know you need to move. You make a deal, as I have said before, where you are moving part of your body now and "Boy," at recess or lunchtime, you are really going to move your body from head to toe.

Crystals are also good to have in your room to ground you.

When you have lots of tears and emotions you need to be grounded so you get to the real problem not just the emotions.

I have an amethyst crystal by my bedside – it makes me feel so good.

An amethyst is also a recharger so, if at school I have had to work my worry stone overtime because my mind just won't settle down, then at night before I go to sleep, I sit my worry stone on the amethyst overnight night, and it gets recharged and ready for the next day.

I have a little list at the back of this book for your mind codes and crystals, along with mind codes and colours to help you out. I thought sometimes mums and dads often find it hard to step out of the norm and out of the square, so you just have to ease them into this new coding system. Once they know the codes, they are right by themselves.

I think in the world today us kids are going to have to be their support as lots of these adults' minds are not working either.

Tip Number 3

Using oils for the mind and body.

Dad really got this one. Just like a Ford Mustang, when the car is not running right, you have to check the oil. Like a squeaky door, if you want it to work, you put some oil on it.

Every oil just like every colour, every number and every crystal has a code. You connect your mind to what is happening to the code of the oil.

Make sure you get pure essential oils. We only buy our oils from the Chris Brazel shop because we know we get the right oil for us.

You can be put in the wrong direction sometimes because someone wants to sell you an oil, but they only want to sell an oil and they are not connected to the codes or the power of the oils.

So, what do you do with the oil?

You have two choices. One you can put it in an oil burner and the smell drifts through your room. Your mind and the room feel amazing.

The second choice is to use it on your body. Just get your mum to check that you do not have any allergies to the oils that you are going to use.

Some oils you can put directly on your hands, wrists, and some you need a carrier oil.

We use the carrier oil most of the time. We use a grapeseed oil.

To mix you simply take a couple of tablespoons of grapeseed oil and put it in a container then put in a few drops of the oil that you need for your mind.

Normally we put the oil on our wrists and rub the two wrists together. The other way is to put it on your hands and rub them together.

The wrists connect to the mind to find which direction you need to go.

The hands connect to receiving.

Both are great.

You can put a little behind your ears if you need to find answers and messages.

Here are a few oils I use. There are heaps more you can learn about.

The best thing, as I tell all my friends who are not onto this easy way to train your brain, kick butt with red flags and medication is to start with the oils you can.

Who wants their mind to turn off when you can simply train your brain and control your mind and your thoughts? A much better way for the future.

The Oils I use:

Bergamot

I use this one either by itself or with the grapeseed oil.
It is great when you need to release a worry, or remove obstacles you feel are in your way, or just let go of a thought that you don't want in your head.

Orange

This oil we always put with grapeseed oil. This is a great oil when you want to be creative with ways of solving problems. It gives you a feeling of joy and that everything will be ok.

Lavender

A healing oil you can either use directly or in the grapeseed oil. It helps to heal and release tension that you may be feeling. It also helps you to relax and be calm and gives you a feeling of peace.

Rose

Rose lifts you up through the energy of your heart. If you are angry, then work with this one. There is no point in being angry. The sooner you let the anger out, the better you will feel.

Rose simply connects to love, and we all need love. When you love yourself, things can start to change. When you make a conscious choice to use this oil you are making a choice that you want and need a little love in your life.

Frankincense

This is a spiritual oil. It is great for cleansing your room or cleaning your mind. This oil I use in a burner and mainly use it in my room.

Never put frankincense on a cut or any damaged skin on your body. I think the best way is to always use this oil in the burner for your room.

Eucalyptus

I like this oil for when I have exams, or my mind is confused. It really helps a foggy mind to start to become clear.

These are my main secret weapons that I have to share with you.

Give them a go. You have nothing to lose and everything to win.

Henry C

Crystals, Special Stones for the Mind

Henry C

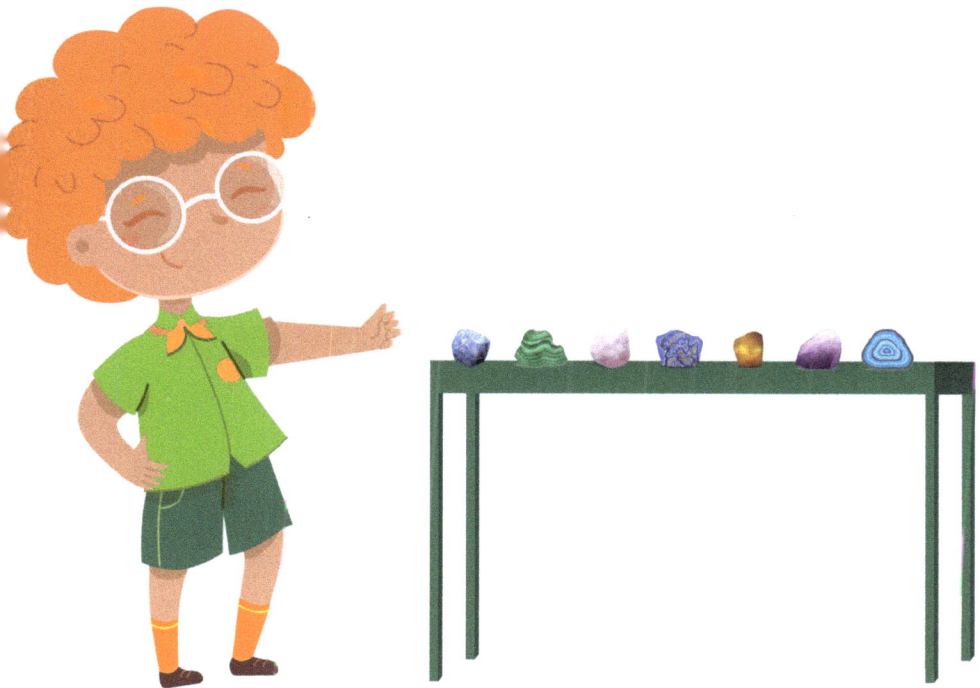

Crystals, Special Stones for the Mind

Crystals are special gems that come from the ground. There are heaps and heaps of crystals to learn about. Every crystal has a special meaning and a special energy.

You just pick the crystal that connects to your brain code or the crystal that gives you the energy connection you need.

Because I have a 1 brain code, amethyst is great for me to meditate with and work with as my secret weapon.

I have a selenite lamp as that connects to my 7 path code which I turn on every night. Selenite is a great crystal to cleanse the mind and give you clarity.

I have a list of crystals below you can check out.

I also have a list of brain codes and the crystal that works with that code.

You have nine brain codes you know.

I will show you how to work with just one. That is your natural code. When you work with your natural code it is the most important code, as that is what your body needs naturally. It is like water. You need water to live, so, when you know your natural code, you know what your brain needs most of all.

Crystals are just helping energy that you can work with.

Here you go. To work out your natural code take the day that you were born.

If you were born on the 1st like me, you will have a brain code of 1 as your natural code.

If you were born on the 12th like one of my friends, you simply take 1+2 = 3. Your natural code is 3.

Here are the crystals to match your natural codes.

Number One	Citrine, Amethyst
Number Two	Moonstone, Tiger Eye
Number Three	Turquoise, Howlite, Amethyst
Number Four	Jade, Aventurine, Rose Quartz
Number Five	Selenite *(a selenite lamp is the best way to work)*
Number Six	Lapis, Malachite
Number Seven	Amethyst, Carnelian, Fluorite
Number Eight	Citrine, Gold Topaz
Number Nine	Garnet, Bloodstone

If you just want to select a crystal for what it can help you with, I have a few below for you to choose from.

The best thing is to go to a crystal shop and just feel the crystals. When you pick one up it will either feel great or not.

Or another way is to get your mum to get in touch with Chris Brazel. Have a chat with her while your mum is there and ask her for the best crystal for you.

She also has prayer beads. They are great. You hold the beads in your hand, and you say the right words for your head. It works all the time.

Now the crystals.

Amethyst

This fixes and works for most things. Helps you to relax and believe in yourself. A healing stone when you feel a little sad.

Rose Quartz

This is a stone that makes you feel calm and at peace. It is a stone that connects to love and we all need a little love.

If you are worried you just take the rose quartz and massage it in your hand. You feel great in no time.

Jade

A feel-good stone and a very lucky stone. If you want to attract a little more luck or pocket money, this is the stone to use.

Malachite

This stone helps you to open the heart and to feel love. Holding the stone in your hand makes you feel strong and safe like being under a tree.

Tiger Eye

This crystal is good when you need to create balance. Sometimes our minds and our body get out of balance.

Hematite

This is an excellent grounding stone. If you feel emotional or have too many thoughts going through your head, then this one will work for you.

This stone helps you feel peace and get back in harmony with your mind and your body.

Bloodstone

This is a great stone to ground you and make you feel protected. I find if I hold it in my hands and I work on my breath I get messages.

It is like the light switch has been turned on and I get an answer to what I have been worried about.

I do find it is a great stone to use if you need a little courage. Maybe courage to speak up. Maybe courage to climb a hill or get through your exams. It is ok to use something like a crystal to get a little courage from time to time.

There are heaps more that you can learn about crystals. I thought I would just help you kick off with a little information. If you want to know more, come join one of our CB Club meetings, which are online, or come to one of our camps where we learn so much.

By the time we leave we have the tools to conquer the world.

I still have lots more to teach you so keep going.

Henry C.

Time Out. Sit and be Still.
Breathe and be at Peace

Henry C

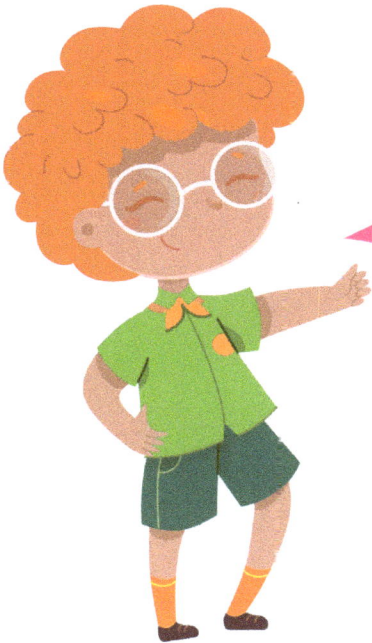

Time Out. Sit and be Still. Breathe and be at Peace

One of my favourite times is to find a tree and just sit under the tree.

Sometimes I lean my back against the tree. Other times I just sit in front of the tree.

When I sit there, I close my eyes and I sit in a yoga pose. I learnt it from my mum.

I then take deep breaths in and out. After a while I then work with the word "Om." I just hum it until my breath runs out.

It is really good. Sometimes I take my crystal and hold it in my hand. Other times I just take my special crystal and have it in my pocket.

I actually prefer to have my crystal in my pocket and sit in the yoga pose with my yoga fingers together. You can give them both a go and see what works for you.

Before I head there, I give either my mum or dad the signage for time out.

They now get it, and they don't disturb me.   Chris Brazel explained that I needed my time out.

It was because I had two 7 codes for my brain. WOW! What a difference it makes when your mum and dad know how your brain works with these codes. It just stops all the hassles and unnecessary arguments.

The reason trees are good to sit under is that the tree can ground you. When your head or mind is all over the place, sitting under a tree or being near a tree is great. Just as the roots of the tree go deep and have stability to grow tall, you can connect to the tree and feel the same energy.

If you need a little more stability in your life, you could put a picture of a tree you love in your bedroom. That will help you feel your bedroom is grounded and you are safe.

I actually don't have a tree picture, but I do have the horse and boy picture from one of Chris Brazel's collections. I love looking at it before I go to sleep – it makes me feel supported and comfortable.

I also have a picture of Mother Mary to whom I pray when I need things and I have God above me to protect me. No sense in having to carry all the worries of life when each night you can hand your worries over to God or Mother Mary.

They both do an amazing job. I always wake up feeling great and ready to take on a new day.

I might add I have another tip for you here.

When you wake up, make sure you say, "Thank you for this new day."

If you say thank you for the day, you are in gratitude. When you are grateful for the little things in your life you get to have more things and bigger things come into your life that you love.

It does not take long, but it is well worth doing. It is really a thought, or you can say the words out loud. I just think it, as that works for me.

Well, that was my last tip for you in creating a great life.

I hope you have enjoyed the journey and my tips help you and your family.

They have certainly helped me, mum and dad.

This is Henry C signing out. I hope to see you one day at a bootcamp, TV session or school camp.

You never know where we may meet.

Henry C

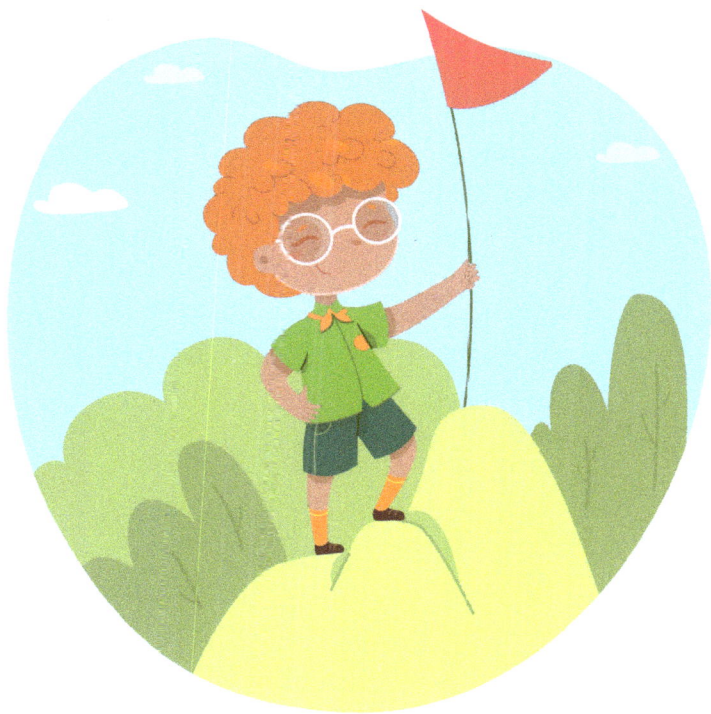

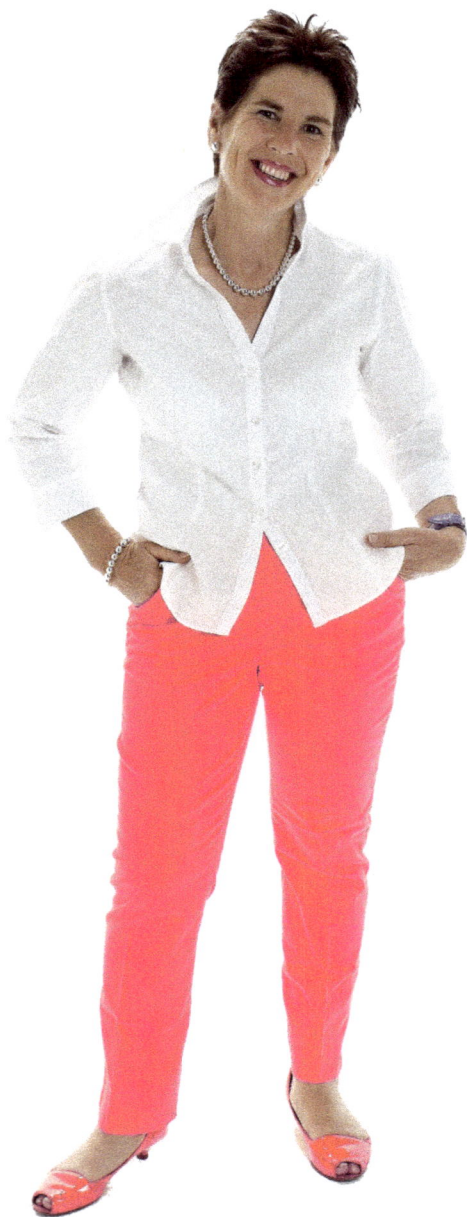

A message direct from Chris Brazel

I loved working with Henry C and his mum and dad.

This is a real boy whom I have worked with and changed his life along with his mum's and dad's life.

Thank you for being part of my world. Come join me for a school camp or an excursion one day. You can even join my CB club and meet me on my YouTube channel.

Always remember everyone is an individual with a unique brain code. Know your brain code and you will know how your mind works and why you do the things you do.

Better still, you will know how to fix the mind when it is not doing what you want it to do.

Chris Brazel

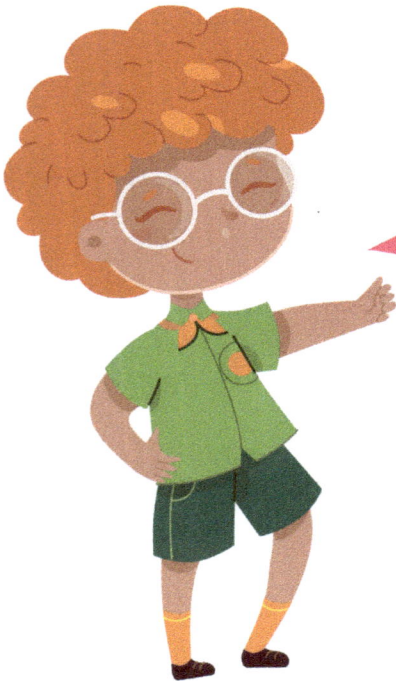

A message
from mum
and me.

A Message from Henry C and his Mum

She understands me from just doing my brain codes. She helped my parents understand me and to listen to me. I kept telling mum my room felt lonely, but nothing got done.

Chris Brazel came over and looked at my bedroom and she had to tell mum it felt lonely. We did the changes, and my room is not lonely anymore.

Chris Brazel taught me about colours and crystals, and she got it right my favourite colour is red.

Chris Brazel was spot on about my timeout and she explained it to my mum. My secret weapons help me during school and the other activities. Chris Brazel has taught me ways to keep me focused.

You are the best Chris Brazel! Thanks for helping us.
Your magic works.

Henry C

I hope this book inspires you to connect with your child and support their needs.

I refused to medicate my child as per a request from a teacher.

I called Chris Brazel as I know how amazing her work is. I have worked with Chris Brazel for many years and whenever I have needed help or a change in our life, she has been able to help us.

I wish you all the success in helping other children be able to know their mind and how their mind works. I do hope other parents start to understand both their own mind and the mind of their child and how the two work as a team.

Thank you, Chris Brazel.

Henry C's Mum

Notes

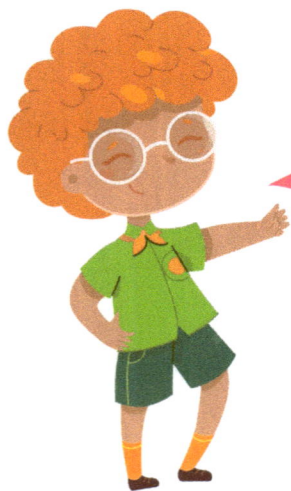

Do you want to write some notes?

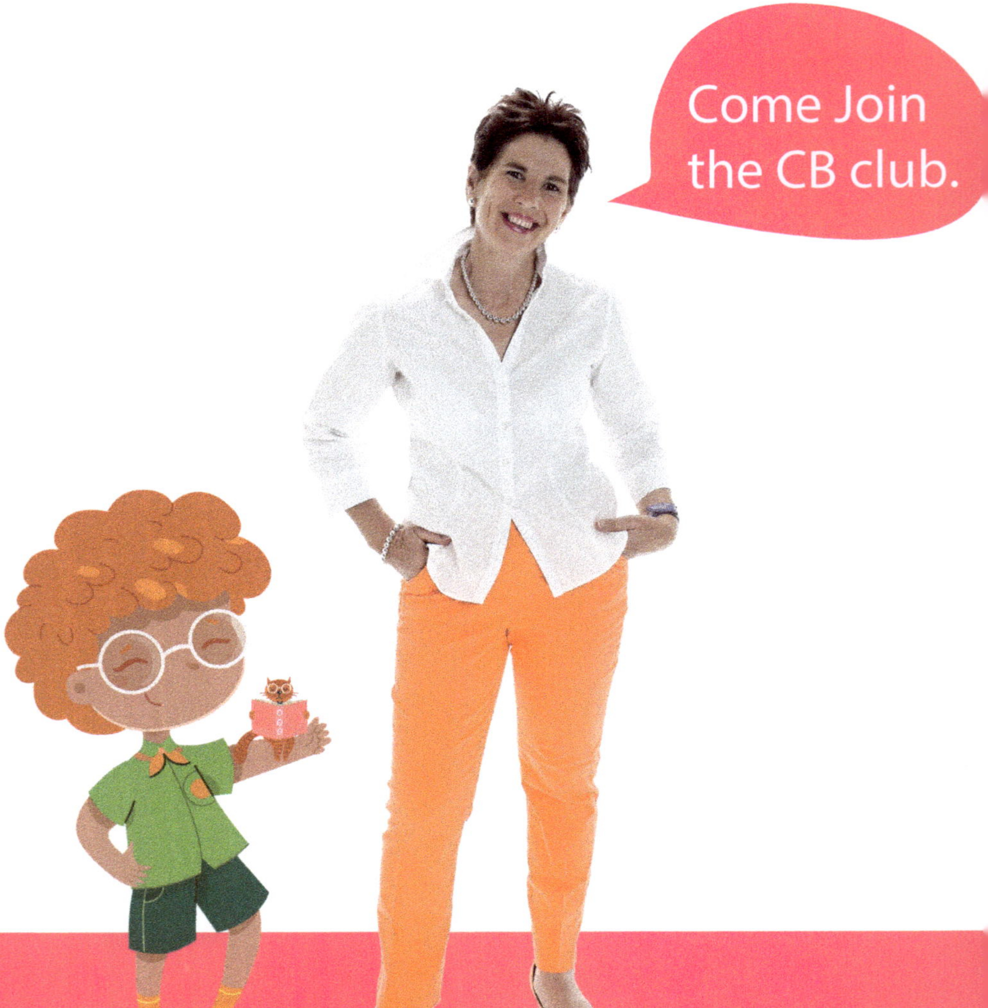

Chris Brazel Products

Check out our website for
artwork, t-shirts, other books.

Join our club or come
join a boot camp.

www.ingramcontent.com/pod-product-compliance
Lightning Source LLC
Chambersburg PA
CBHW041301040426
42334CB00028BA/3113